© Copyright 2018 by - All rights reserved.

The following eBook is reproduced below with the goal of providing information that is as accurate and reliable as possible. Regardless, purchasing this eBook can be seen as consent to the fact that both the publisher and the author of this book are in no way experts on the topics discussed within and that any recommendations or suggestions that are made herein are for entertainment purposes only. Professionals should be consulted as needed prior to undertaking any of the action endorsed herein.

This declaration is deemed fair and valid by both the American Bar Association and the Committee of Publishers Association and is legally binding throughout the United States.

Furthermore, the transmission, duplication or reproduction of any of the following work including specific information will be considered an illegal act irrespective of if it is done electronically or in print. This extends to creating a secondary or tertiary copy of the work or a recorded copy and is only allowed with an express written consent from the Publisher. All additional rights reserved.

The information in the following pages is broadly considered to be a truthful and accurate account of facts and as such any inattention, use or misuse of the information in question by the reader will render any resulting actions solely under their purview. There are no scenarios in which the publisher or the original author of this work can be in any fashion deemed liable for any hardship or damages that may befall them after undertaking information described herein.

Additionally, the information in the following pages is intended only for informational purposes and should thus be thought of as universal. As befitting its nature, it is presented without assurance regarding its prolonged validity or interim quality. Trademarks that are mentioned are done without written consent and can in no way be considered an endorsement from the trademark holder.

Contents

Chapter 1: What The F*%k Is Intermittent Fasting?

Intermittent fasting is the term used to describe eating patterns that involves cycles between eating and fasting. It is not considered to be a "diet" since it's not about selecting certain foods and more about time intervals between meals.

Many people adopt the method of doing 16 to 24 hour fasts a couple of times per week. Relatively longer time intervals between meals were a way of life that humans adapted to in the past since food was not readily available as it is for most of us in the 21st century. Some cultures and religions practiced fasting in the past including Christianity, Islam, Judaism, and Buddhism.

It can be argued that fasting is even more natural than eating several meals each day. Imagine living in the ancient times where there were no supermarkets, refrigerators, or restaurants that give us food on demand, whenever we feel like it. People didn't have access to an abundance of food all year round so our bodies have evolved and adapted to cope without food for long periods of time.

It might seem odd to think that depriving yourself from the food, a key necessity to life, can powerfully transform one's health. However, the health benefits are well documented and the evidence seems to be growing as more studies are conducted. The brain and body tend to benefit from the fasting process. In fact, celebrities including Hugh Jackman, Tim Ferriss, and Beyoncé are believers in intermittent fasting.

Throughout Silicon Valley, the 'biohackers' who do everything within their power to optimize their health and performance, experiment with smart drugs and nootropics, and on top of that implement a routine that includes intermittent fasting. This allows people to bypass the 'food comas' and conserve the mental energy wasted on deciding where the next meal will come from. This allows its participants to stay focused and productive all day.

How To Practice Intermittent Fasting

There are different methods when it comes to intermittent fasting. They usually involve splitting the day or week into separate "eating periods" and "fasting periods". In the fasting periods you either eat nothing or very little.

Common methods include:

Eat-stop-eat: This is where you fast for 24 hours for one or two times per week.

The 16/8 Method: this is where you choose an 8-hour period to eat in, outside of this time interval you will fast. For instance, you might choose to eat only between this hours of 12pm to 8pm, and then in the remaining 16 hours you will fast.

The 5:2 Diet: This is where on two non-consecutive days each week you only eat between 500 and 600 calories (2100 – 2500 kilojoules)

By lowering one's calorie intake consistently the probability of losing weight significantly increase assuming that you don't eat an excess in the periods where you can eat.

Some people argue that the 16/8 method is the easiest to stick to which is why it is the most popular. It's worth experimenting and seeing which technique works best for you.

How Intermittent Fasting Affects the Cells and Hormones

When we fast, a myriad of changes start to take place within the body on a molecular to cellular level.

For instance, our body changes its hormone levels to allow for stored body fat to be more accessible.

Our cells also initiate the processes that are responsible for repairing the body as well as the expression of our genes.

When we fast, the following changes tend to occur:

Human Growth Hormone: Our levels of growth hormone rise sharply, increasing by up to 5 times. Higher HGH levels are correlated with higher levels of lean muscle mass – meaning more muscle and less fat.

Cellular repair: During a fast, the cells initiate cellular repair process. This process is known as autophagy. Cells digest and remove old and dysfunctional proteins that build up within the cell.

Insulin: Our insulin sensitivity improves which causes the insulin levels to drop. When our insulin levels are lower, stored body fat becomes more accessible.

Gene expression: Changes to the function of our genes take place which have been correlated with longevity and protection against disease(11, 12)

These key changes improve our hormone levels, cell functions, and gene expressions which improve our health and help us lose body fat.

Autophagy

"Our food should be our medicine. Our medicine should be our food. But to eat when you are sick is to feed your sickness."

- Hippocrates of Ancient Greece, the "Father of Western Medicine"

The body is a genius that is self-repairing. One of the key processes in the body that facilitates the healing process is known as Autophagy. In this chapter we will dive deeply into the biological processes associated with autophagy.

Autophagy is derived from the Ancient Greek word "autophagos" which means "self-devouring". Autophagy is described by scientists as "The body's innate recycling program". It helps to stop cancerous growths by removing faulty cells and regulate insulin levels which help to prevent metabolic dysfunctions such as obesity and diabetes.

Simply put, autophagy is a self-digesting process that allows for the removal or malformed proteins, damaged organelles, and non-functional long-lived proteins. There are three forms of autophagy, which are macroautophagy, microautophagy, and chaperone-mediated autophagy.

All types of autophagy have one common feature which is the degradation of substrates within the lysosome, the breakdown of proteins, lipid droplets, or organelles. It is responsible for cellular waste clearance, including the recycling of nutrient subunits except amino acids. Autophagy also helps to promote homeostasis, which is essentially physiological equilibrium – the balancing of the body's biochemistry in order to achieve a stable state which results in optimal functioning.

Macroautophagy

Macroautophagy is an umbrella term that covers the various types of macoautophagies, including mitophagy, reticulophagy, nucleophagy lipophagy, and xenophagy. These processes help to prevent cancer, Crohn's disease, neurodegeneration, and metabolic diseases.

Microautophagy

Microautophagy is important for the survival of cells under starvation. There are three types of selective microautophagy: macropexophagy, piecemeal microautophagy of the nucleus, and micro mitophagy.

Chaperone-Mediated Autophagy

Chaperone-mediated autophagy is where cytosolic proteins are degraded after reaching the cytosol. CMA helps to maintain the cellular homeostasis by assisting in the recycling of amino acids that are derived from the degraded proteins. CMA is an active process that is taking place at all times, however its process is quickened as a response to limitations in nutrient supplies i.e fasting.

How To Enable The Autophagic Process

Regular exercise is a powerful means of facilitating the autophagy process. This is arguably why we experience a fresh clean feeling after undergoing rigorous exercise. A study done on mice which involved genetically engineering them to have glowing green autophagosomes, scientists found that the rate that the mice were healthily eliminating unneeded cells at a significantly faster rate than normal after just 30 minutes of exercise. The rate consistently increased until they had been running for 80 minutes.

Eating ironically halts the process of autophagy. Skipping meals however, works incredibly well. Many studies have shown that fasting promotes autophagy in the brain, which suggests that it could be an effective technique for mitigating the risks associated with neurodegenerative diseases such as Alzheimer's and Parkinson's.

Scientific and anecdotal evidence support a vast array of benefits from fasting when compared to consistent eating.

Once you have calculated your macronutrient requirements for cutting weight, dieting becomes easier. For losing weight, less emphasis can be placed on what you eat and more on the quantities consumed. You can enjoy your favourite foods when the temptations arise. As we can see, losing weight is achievable when consuming almost any food types, however it is still more beneficial to aim for a diet that is rich in whole foods to avoid vitamin deficiencies.

Fasting and BDNF

Brain-Derived Neurotrophic factor or "BDNF" is the term used for describing a naturally occurring growth hormone that is required for the process of neurogenesis – the formation of new neurons.

Higher levels of BDNF are correlated with increases in intelligence, memory, mood, and productivity. BDNF has been found to lower the chances of developing neurodegenerative such as Alzheimer's and Parkinson's.

BDNF is believed to contain "a crucial biological link between, thoughts, emotions, and movement," according to John J. Ratey, an associate professor from Harvard Medical School. He then went on to say that, "Physical exercise is really for our brains. It turns our brains on." Ratey also calls BDNF "miracle grow for the brain" (*miracle grow* is a popular fertilizer).

Art De Vany, an "evolutionary fitness expert" made an interesting statement about BDNF.

"When BDNF is released, new connections form in the brain as the BDNF attracts new dendrites from nerve cells to connect to other cells or their synapses. As the brain cells "fire together", they "wire together." Wiring together new networks is how memory is formed and consolidated. A neural network is a thought, a memory, or a new skill. This "fast" form of learning is essential in emergency situations where fight or flight may be the only means of coping. Evolution would seem to require that fast learning takes precedence in fight or flight situations and the release of BDNF and stress hormones during such episodes almost assures that the event takes on salience and weight."

So as well as exercise, how else can we increase our BDNF?

Lower our sugar intake

Diets that are high in sugar reduce our BDNF levels. So, by avoiding processed foods, refined sugars, eating whole foods, and limiting caloric intake, you give yourself a higher probability of achieving optimal brain function.

Sprints

A number of studies have supported the link between high intensity training and increases in BDNF and cognition.

Sprints were shown increase learning abilities by 20% when compared with low intensity exercise or rest.

The participants in the study showed improvements in their vocabularies.

The high intensity exercise routine that was considered to be responsible for this improvement was a 3 minute sprint followed by a 2 minute rest, which was then followed by another 3 minute sprint.

High Intensity Resistance Training

It's important to remember the nature of our biology,
millions of years of natural selection have supported
the most adaptable of beings, able to run, jump, and
fight.

In a way, that is what we were designed to do. A
lifestyle without intensive exercise is neglecting the
nature of our body. It shouldn't be a surprise that
intensive exercise equips us for success, making us
smarter and more adaptable.

Why Intermittent Fasting Is Great For Losing Weight

The main reason people try with intermittent fasting is to lose weight. (13)

Reducing the amount of meals consumed each day generally lowers one's calorie intake.

Fasting has been practiced by humans for thousands of years, and is a prescribed practice in many religions, for example, Catholic Christians practice lent, and Muslims observe Ramadan. Modern medicine has studied prolonged fasting as a way of achieving weight loss since the early 1900s. While initial studies on fasting supported the technique as a safe and effective tool for weight loss, interest in the subject quickly faded away.

Interest was revived in the late 1950s. Studies initially focused on shorter fasting periods, but as research progressed, scientists eventually began to extend the length of the fasts.

Ian Gilliland, an endocrinologist, studied the effects of fasting for an extended period in a study set in a hospital to monitor the conditions of the patients. The forty-six patients were only allowed to drink water, tea, or coffee over the fourteen-day fasting period, and then following that they were prescribed a 600 to 1000 calorie a day diet after they were sent home from the hospital. The results were extremely positive. In fact, two patients even asked to undergo the treatment again as they wanted to continue to achieve the results that the treatment provided.

Patients in the study lost weight at an average of 17.2 pounds per patient. But the effects of fasting were not limited to only weight loss. The diabetic patients that participated in the trial no longer required insulin by the end of the two-week fasting period, as their blood sugar levels had fell significantly to levels at which the patient no longer required medication to regulate their condition. A patient who had experienced severe congestive heart failure experienced significant improvements and was able to walk without breathlessness after the treatment due to the effect of fasting. This was due to an effect experienced during the first few days of fasting, where an increased urine flow eliminates excess water and salt from the kidneys. Patients described enjoying the treatment, experiencing feelings of well-being and euphoria. Hunger complaints were non-existent after the first day, which was an effect that is commonly noted in fasting research.

Gilliland's study was one of many which showed significant positive health benefits for fasting as a tool for weight loss. Not only were the health benefits apparent, but patient's mental health also improved. These studies provide a strong case for the practice of fasting.

Intermittent fasting alters our hormone levels, which makes our body more inclined to losing body fat.

The lowered insulin levels and increases in growth hormone triggers the release of the fat burning hormone known as norepinephrine. These hormone changes caused from short-term fasting can increase one's metabolic rate by 3.6 to 14 percent. (14, 15).

By eating less, we prevent weight gain and allow our body to burn fat at an even faster rate, influencing both sides of the calorimetric equation.

Studies have shown that intermittent fasting can function as a very effective weight loss tool. In a study conducted in 2014, intermittent fasting was shown to cause weight loss ranging from 3 to 8 percent reductions over a 3 to 24-week interval. (1).

This is a significant amount of weight loss compared to the vast majority of weight loss studies.

Another study showed that people last between 4 and 7 percent of their waist circumference. (1). This means that the participants lost a large amount of harmful belly fat which tends to build up around the organs and cause disease.

Studies have also shown that intermittent fasting results in less muscle loss than the conventional method of calorie restriction. (16).

It is important to note that the key reason intermittent fasting works is because of the lowered calorie intake. If one is to eat in excess during the eating periods, then the chances of losing weight is reduced. Losing weight is simple but limiting one's calorie intake tends to be the main challenge for the average person.

How The Body Benefits From Intermittent Fasting

Studies have been conducted on both animals and humans for intermittent fasting. The results are astonishing, intermittent fasting has been shown to do more than just help us lose weight: its been shown to have anti-aging effects as well as increase longevity.

The key benefits that have been explored include:

Weight loss: Intermittent fasting can help us lose weight and belly fat.(1, 13).

Insulin resistance: Intermittent fasting tends to reduce insulin resistance, lowers blood sugar by 3-6 percent

which functions as a preventative for type 2 diabetes.
(1)

Heart Health: Intermittent fasting is good for the heart since inflammatory markers, blood triglycerides, blood sugar, and insulin resistance are all correlated with heart disease.

Cancer: Animal studies have shown that intermittent fasting can help prevent the growth of cancers. (22, 23, 24, 25)

Inflammation: Studies show that intermittent fasting lowers inflammation throughout the body which is vital since inflammation is known to be a driver of chronic disease.

Brain: There is a brain hormone called BDNF which intermittent fasting increases. The BDNF hormone can aid in the growth of new nerve cells and also protect against Alzheimer's disease. (26, 27, 28) (29).

Anti-aging: In a study conducted on rats, intermittent fasting was shown that rats live as much as 36-83% longer than rats that are able to eat at will.

It is worth noting that many of these studies are still in their early stages. The studies were short and done over small periods of time and often on animals. There are still many questions yet to be answered. (32).

10 Benefits of Intermittent Fasting.

How Fasting Affects The Heart

Throughout our lives, we have been taught general guidelines for how to take care of our body by our parents and society. For example, having three meals a day is not always necessary, but that's how we've been taught to eat. From the study of fasting, we have learned that what we've been taught about our bodies might not always be correct. Another 'myth' that we've been taught is that high blood cholesterol is bad for the health of our hearts, increasing our risk for heart attacks and strokes. This 'myth' isn't completely untrue. Some types of cholesterol is bad for you. However, to say that all types of cholesterol is bad for you is a lie.

Cholesterol's role in your body is to repair damage in cells, and to produce certain hormones. Every cell in the body can make cholesterol, as it is vital to our health. There are two types of cholesterol, low-density lipoprotein (LDL), or high-density lipoprotein (HDL). The main cholesterol molecule is the same in both types, however as the cholesterol travels through the bloodstream it becomes associated with different proteins. LDL is considered the 'bad' type of cholesterol - the molecules are bigger, as the proteins take up more space. This can cause blockages in the arteries. HDL is considered 'good' protein as it completes its role of cell repair and hormone production without restricting blood flow. While high levels of LDL in the bloodstream can be treated using statins, the root cause of the problem must be treated. Unlike other health factors for heart disease, such as high levels of a type of fat called triglycerides which can be moderated through diet, high levels of LDL is not exactly a dietary issue.

In the last few decades, we have been told by health-care professionals to eat less high-cholesterol foods, such as egg yolks as they reasoned that eating more cholesterol would raise blood cholesterol levels. It was believed that high blood cholesterol levels would cause an increased risk in heart disease. However, as LDL and HDL was identified, it was clear that it wasn't the cholesterol level in the blood that caused heart disease, it was the density of the proteins attaching to the cholesterol molecules. The liver creates most of the cholesterol in the body, and compensates whenever the body receives too much or little outside sources of cholesterol, so diet has an almost negligible effect on your body's cholesterol levels.

The fear of cholesterol started with the discovery that blockages in the arteries that lead to heart attacks and strokes were made of cholesterol, and the natural conclusion was that cholesterol caused these blockages. However, later studies found that the level of cholesterol intake had little to no effect on blood cholesterol. While the other obvious solution would be that it was the dietary intake of fat that increased the risk of heart disease, this was also later disproven. Decades of society following these disproven practices have millions of people today still partaking in low-fat, low-cholesterol diet plans despite their ineffectiveness in creating any significant health benefits.

When you fast, the liver begins to receive less dietary carbohydrates, which in turn causes it to produce less triglycerides. As there are less triglycerides in the blood, less LDL is produced. Studies have consistently shown that fasting can cause a significant decrease in blood LDL. Fasting has been shown to be more effective than statin medication, which means patients can achieve better results fasting without the risk of diabetes or Alzheimer's disease associated with statin use. While fasting lowers LDL, HDL levels are maintained. Overall, fasting provides many health benefits for the heart, and can replace many of the practices we currently use. Instead of medication or diet modification, a simple fast can be all we need.

Your Muscles During Fasting

You are probably not going to gain muscle during your fasting period. In order to gain muscle, you must have an excess supply of calories and protein, and also exercise. During fasting your excess supply of calories is easily depleted during exercise and it is difficult to have enough readily available protein. However, while muscle gain is difficult during fasting, maintenance of your current muscle mass and strength can be achieved through weight training.

Studies into intermittent fasting have shown that when controlling for exercise and amount of calories and protein consumed each day, people who are fasting are able to maintain the same lean mass as those who were not, while still being able to lose fat mass. There were no losses in strength or muscle mass in the fasting groups. In order to maintain muscle mass, a steady intake of protein is usually recommended. While longer term studies document the effects of weight and fat loss in the study's participants, they rarely focus on the effects on the muscles. However the data suggests that muscle mass is generally maintained as long as there is exercise. Extreme muscle loss effects are rarely documented, except in cases of severe long term starvation, which is different to fasting.

Research into the effects of fasting on muscles has focused more on intermittent fasting, where the fasting period is usually less than 48 hours. When combating muscle loss, it is suggested to focus on not losing weight too fast. A diet high in protein is also prescribed, as this can help significantly in maintaining muscle mass. During feeding periods, some supplements may also help in muscle retention, for example, creatine. However, other supplements could have undesired effects, for example amino acid supplements during fasting can indicate to the body that it is still feeding. With all that said, studies have not shown fasting to cause significant muscle loss, especially in short term fasting, so most people should just focus on maintaining an adequate exercise routine during their fasting periods.

Just like with everything else associated with fasting, society has misguided us on the effect of fasting on muscles. It is commonly thought that once the body runs out of energy stores, it will start to consume itself and its muscles for energy, and this process begins soon after a person stops eating. This effect is seen in severely malnourished people. However, the majority of us are well nourished, and have plenty of fat stored for energy. Someone who is used to having 3 meals a day should not worry about muscle loss during a short term fast. Fasting is not recommended for somebody who is already malnourished.

Let Intermittent Fasting Simplify Your Life

Intellectually, eating healthy is simple, but it's still quite tricky to stick to.

One of the key challenges is allocating time to prepare and cook healthy meals. Intermittent fasting makes this simple as it doesn't require time to prepare, cook, and clean up the dishes.

Intermittent fasting is popular among the hyper efficient lifehacker types since it improves your health and frees up time.

People Who Should Be Mindful About Intermittent Fasting Or Avoid It Altogether

Not everyone should be doing intermittent fasting. If you are underweight or have a history of eating disorders then it should be avoided unless you seek advice from a health professional.

For some people intermittent fasting can be harmful.

Should Women Fast?

Some evidence has suggested that intermittent fasting is more beneficial for men than women.

There was a study that showed that it improved insulin sensitivity in men but negatively altered blood sugar control in women (33).

A study on rats found that fasting can make female rats scrawny, infertile, and even miss menstrual cycles. (34, 35).

Some women have reported having inconsistent menstrual cycles which returned to normal once moving back to their old diet.

Because of these concerns women should be careful with intermittent fasting. Start with the least intensive routine and if you have any problems such as amenorrhea (irregular menstrual cycles) then revert to consistent eating.

If you have having problems with fertility, trying to conceive, are pregnant, or breastfeeding it is probably a good idea to avoid intermittent fasting.

Side Effects and Safety

For the most part, hunger is the key side effect of intermittent fasting. You may also feel as though your brain isn't performing as efficiently and you might feel weak. These are the main initial effects which will subside once your body becomes accustomed to intermittent fasting.

If you have any medical conditions or are on any medications, then it's safer to speak with your doctor before experimenting with intermittent fasting.

This is especially important if you suffer from one or more of the following conditions:

- Diabetes.

- Issues with blood sugar regulation.

    Low blood pressure.

Once again if you are having inconsistent menstrual cycles, fertility issues, pregnant or breastfeeding avoid intermittent fasting.

In saying this, intermittent fasting has an exceptionally safety profile. There shouldn't be any danger in not eating for a while if you are healthy and well nourished for the most part – remember, our ancestors likely went for very long periods of time without food.

Refeeding Syndrome

Refeeding syndrome is a rare condition which occurs due to a depletion in phosphorus and magnesium in the body. People who are at risk of refeeding syndrome are typically already malnourished previous to fasting, such as people with drug addictions or anorexia. Generally, people who are fasting for weight loss are not at risk of refeeding syndrome.

The body stores a limited amount of phosphorus in the body, which is to maintain the healthy condition of bones in the body. When the body begins to refeed, insulin levels are raised, which begins the production of glycogen, fat, and protein, all molecules that require phosphorus and magnesium. As phosphorus stores are continually used up and not recycled, this additional demand severely depletes the body's stores and can cause muscle weakness, or even muscle breakdown. This damage can extend to vital muscle organs, such as the heart. Magnesium depletion results in cramps, tremors, and seizures. The increase in insulin can also increase water retention, resulting in swelling of the limbs.

People who are underweight or who are at risk of being malnourished through fasting should not attempt medium or long term fasting. Short term fasts will not cause the effects of refeeding syndrome. Even so, refeeding syndrome is rare.

If there is a reason to fast even with the risk of refeeding syndrome, it is recommended that the fast is supplemented with a bone soup broth, as this will help replenish essential phosphorus and other building blocks. Exercise during the fasting period is also prescribed to maintain healthy bones. The key to avoid refeeding syndrome is to not take extremes. An

extended fast is a tool to lose weight, which a person

with a healthy weight should not use inappropriately.

Getting Started

There are no technical skills needed to begin intermittent fasting. It is highly likely that you have already completed many "intermittent fasts" throughout your life. If you have ever eaten dinner, then slept in until lunch time then you have likely already done a 16 hour or greater fast. Some people intermittently fast on a regular basis, unknowingly. They don't feel hungry in the mornings, so they skip breakfast.

The 16/8 method is the simplest and easiest method to follow and it is recommended that you try that one first.

If the 16/8 fast feels easy and you are satisfied with the way you feel then you can try experimenting with the more advanced fasts. This could include 24 hour fasts or 500-600 calorie days once or twice each week.

Intermittent fasting can be done whenever you feel is most convenient. Skip meals when you feel like it. Learn to appreciate the times when you are missing meals and feeling hungry, because these times can be used to be ultra-productive. Have you ever noticed that right after eating a meal you feel tired and drained? That's because blood is flowing from the brain to the digestive system and our energy is used to break down food.

A structured intermittent fasting plan is not essential to still achieve some benefits. Experiment with different approaches and listen to your body; see what works best for you.

Is Intermittent Fasting Right For You?

Intermittent fasting isn't essential for living a healthy life, it is not something that everyone has to do. It is simply one of the many strategies that can be adopted to improve one's health. Eating natural food instead of processed ingredients, exercising, and getting regular sleep are cornerstones of living a healthy well balanced life. If your body or nerves are ever feeling out of kilter, make sure these areas are looked after before considering things like anti-depressants.

There is no one size fits all when it comes to nutrition. There is no best diet. Everything must be analysed on a case by case basis – the best diet is one that makes you feel great and one that you are happy to stick to in the long term.

Intermittent fasting is not for everyone, but it is worth experimenting with to see if it works for you. You might find out very early into your fasts that you feel more energized and clear headed on it along with increases in efficiency. After all, it is a tremendously powerful technique for cutting weight.

Top Fasting Tips:

1. Drink a lot of water. Drinking a lot of water is something we should be doing already, but the best

benefit of water during a fast is that it helps take away some of the feelings of hunger. Feelings of hunger are often a result of dehydration and thirst, rather than real hunger.

2. Keep yourself occupied. The first couple of days will pass quickly if you can keep yourself busy during this period. Try to fast on a work day.

3. Enjoy the extra time. As it turns out, eating is a very time-consuming task, especially if you are buying groceries and cooking meals yourself. Also, you won't have to clean! Use the time and reward yourself with an activity that you enjoy.

4. Be resilient. The hunger will be distracting, and may cause you to want to eat to end it. Drink some water, tea, or coffee, and the hunger will pass. Remember, it gets easier after the second day.

5. Drink coffee. Coffee will help suppress your appetite. Bone broth or tea may also help.

6. Keep trying. It will take some time to get used to fasting on a regular schedule, but it gets easier.

7. Eat good food. When you aren't fasting, don't binge on unhealthy foods. A good diet will help maintain the results you gain with fasting.

8. Eat normally. After fasting, just eat as you usually would as if the fast had never happened (though hopefully with a healthier menu!).

9. Don't tell anyone. Our culture has set meal times, and many people think that fasting is a behaviour that will damage your body. It is best to focus on the task yourself, as this is not the time to educate others about your health.

10. Make fasting part of your lifestyle. It's important to remember to still live out your life, and there are plenty of times where fasting is not preferable, such as celebrations or holidays. Also, long term fasts may restrict you from certain activities that you wish to participate in. Fasting as part of your lifestyle is a much more maintainable practice than going to extremes, and balance is required if you want to live life to the fullest. Fast, but adjust your schedule to fit your life.

11. Pay attention. Become aware of your mind and your body. It is up to you to decide whether you think the food craving is a result of a food addiction, emotional triggers, or even dehydration. By consistently applying the principles you have learned in this book, you will begin to be able to distinguish between these

experiences and maintain a state of being satisfied, instead of constantly craving food.

12. Maintain a focus on your goals and vision. You read this book for a reason, because you are ready to make your body's health a priority. Go to the mirror and ask yourself if the snack or cheat meal was really worth it.

13. When a craving comes up, set your timer on your phone to 20 minutes, wait for the time to pass and you will able to see whether the craving was an emotional need or an actual craving.

14. Eat slowly. By eating slowly you are less likely using food as a form of escapism. Chew your food before swallowing. Often it takes time for us to notice when are full which is why eating till we feel a stomach ache is common. The benefits of eating slower has been shown to improve bowel

movements, digestion, and short/long term satiation.

15. Eat without distractions from electronics. Studies have shown that eating while distracted can result in us overeating and feeling less satisfied afterwards.

16. Implement strict kitchen hours. Do not eat outside of designated times. 11am to 8pm can be an ideal range.

17. Do some quick sets of exercise. Push ups, squats, wall sits, or jumping jacks will distract you from your hunger as well as stimulate the body in a way that will resolve the feeling of hunger. A quick intense burst of exercise will also boost your metabolism so that when you do eat, the consequences are less of an impact.

18. Throw out all sugary foods, so that when you do get food cravings the worst-case scenario is that you end up snacking on healthy foods.

Chapter 3: Nutrition & Flexible Dieting

Introduction to Flexible Dieting

The idea of flexible dieting is to eat to an extent whatever food you want. So, for example, you don't need to restrict your diet at social events or at the workplace. The key theme for flexible dieting is tracking your "macros".

What Are Macros?

The foods we eat can be compartmentalized in three categories. The macros include, protein, fat, and carbohydrates.

Macro counting is a powerful way for losing weight, it can also free us from the stress of worrying about whether what we are eating is good or not. You don't have to deprive yourself from your favourite foods in order to lose weight. Ensure that you are measuring your macro counts each day and you are ready to start losing weight!

In general, flexible dieting consists of three steps:

1) Figuring out your Total Daily Energy Expenditure (TDEE) by measuring your current weight and level of exercise.

2) Calculate your macro in ratio requirements in order to reach your desired goal.

3) Monitor your food intake and aim to meet your total energy expenditure and macro limits on a daily basis.

Chapter 4: Calculating Your Macros

How to Count Your Macros

Macronutrients make up the vast majority of our diets.

One gram of every protein, fat, or carbohydrate has a calorie proportion.

1 gram of fat contains 9 calories

1 gram of carbohydrate contains 4 calories

1 gram of protein contains 4 calories

Instead of typical counting, flexible dieters place more emphasis on tracking the macros.

A flexible dieting plan might look like this:

160g Protein

90g Fat

160g Carbohydrate

Flexible dieting is based around the idea that there are no secret weight-loss foods. Losing weight is entirely predicated on macro ratios and energy burnt.

For example, in terms of weight loss goals, there is virtually no difference is outcomes when choosing between the following:

Chicken Burger

30 grams of Protein

35 grams of Carbohydrate

17g grams of Fat

Tuna with Brown Rice

30 grams of Protein

35 grams of Carbohydrate

17g grams of Fat

Both meals have the same macros, which means that the body will experience the same level of weight loss.

When food reaches our stomach, our body isn't judging whether the food is healthy or not, it is simply breaking down what it can. If we want to change our body, it's completely fine eating whatever you want, but it should still coincide with your macro goals.

It is also worth tracking your fibre intake as a means of maintaining and improving overall health. By doing this it will ensure that you are meeting your micronutrient needs. The American Heart Association recommends an intake of 14 grams of fibre for every 1,000 calories consumed.

A good rule of thumb for maintaining good health is to aim to have a diet of at least 80% whole foods (non-processed). This will give you some room for some freedom at things like social events where there aren't any "healthy" options.

So now that the concept of macro nutrients are understood, how do we figure out the right amount of macros for weight loss?

Before one can make sense of the specific requirements for fat loss, flexible dieting needs to be attempted. So, this is where you pick and track your own foods to reach your macronutrient targets, firstly by calculating your calorie target. It is important to note that whatever approach you take when doing calculations, the calorie target is an estimation and not an exact number.

Even if you follow all of the steps, the calculation will still only be an estimation, some modifications may be needed for better results. It can be handy to connect with a nutrition coach who can do the tweaking for you.

There are several ways to calculate/estimate the caloric requirements for weight loss. Here we will be discussing a more complicated and arguably more accurate version rather than just multiplying body weight by a factor like many people do.

Before we start let's look at an example.

Meet Greg. He is a 31-year-old man. He weighs 82kg and is 181cm tall. He lifts weights twice a week and during the day he works his office job – now he wants to analyse his macro requirements for weight loss.

First, we can use the Mifflin-St Jeor formula as a means of estimating his Basal Metabolic Rate (BMR). This is an approximation for the amount of energy expended each day before we factor in energy consumed from physical activity.

The American Dietetic Association (ADA) conducted a study that found the Mifflin-St Jeor method to be quite accurate.

For women: 10 x weight (kg) + 6.25 x height (cm) – 5 x age (years) - 161

For men: 10 x weight (kg) +6.25 x height (cm) – 5 x age (years) + 5

So, for Greg, aged 31 who weighed in at 82kg and 181cm in height, would apply the formula as follows:

(10 x 82) + (6.25 x 181) – (5 x 31) +5 = 1801.25

The Physical Activity Ratio

Since we have figured out Greg's BMR, now it's time to calculate the Physical Activity Ratio which is an estimation measure of activity done each day.

So now Greg will have to multiply the BMR by one of the following:

1.2 If he does little or no exercise

1.4 If he does exercise a couple of time per week

1.5 to 1.7 if he does exercise several times each week

1.9+ if he does exercise every day or has a physical demanding job

Because Greg trains a couple of times each week, we can multiply his BMR(1801.25) by 1.4. This gives an estimation of this Total Daily Energy Expenditure (TDEE) would come to 2521.75

If Greg is serious about losing weight he will need to create a calorie deficit.

He will need to consume less calories than he needs per day as a means of losing weight.

A deficit of approximately 15 percent is a good place to start. There are many cases where we may need to go lower or higher depending on each persons starting body fat levels, goals and also energy requirements.

Nonetheless Greg's calorie target for getting rid of fat would be 2144 calories (TDEE x 0.85).

So now that we know the suitable range of calories to aim for, let's calculate the macro requirements for cutting.

How To Calculate Your Protein Targets?

A diet that is high in protein is an excellent tool for fat loss. Protein helps to preserve and repair muscle tissue as well as keeping us feel fuller for longer.

A good guideline to follow when flexible dieting is to aim for around 2 grams of protein for each kilogram of bodyweight.

So for Greg, 162 grams each day would be a good place to start.

Consuming this much protein in a day can be tricky for some. Protein shakes can be a wonderful way to reach these levels of intake.

How To Calculate Your Fat Targets?

Now we arrive at a topic that leaves many of us curious - how much fat should we be eating?

Fat has a bad reputation. People tend to assume that fat is the worst thing one can eat, which isn't necessarily true. Fat plays an important role in our physiology. Fats are a vital part of our diet and should not be neglected. In fact the brain's circuitry is comprised of many fats and lipids. Within the brain, our neurons are covered in myelin, which acts as a form of insulation to ensure electrical conductivity throughout the nervous system. Myelin is mostly comprised of lipids. Fats are essential for cell growth, repair, and a range of vital bodily functions.

A range of anywhere between 0.7 grams to 1.2 grams of fat for each kg of body mass is a good place to start. So for Greg, approximately 80 grams of fat would be good for him.

How To Calculate Your Carbohydrate Targets?

So far, we have worked out Greg's daily calorie target: 2143 calories

His protein target is 162 grams each day and his fat target is 80 grams each day.

Remember earlier whe we discussed the ratio of 4 calories per gram of protein and 9 calories for each gram of fat. Now to figure out what the carbohydrate intake should be, we can do the following.

(162 x 4) + (80 x 9) = 1368 kcal,

If we subtract 1368 from his calorie target of 2143 he is left with 775 kcal remaining for his carbohydrate intake.

So, we divided this number by 4, since 4kcal per g of carbohydrate is required which leaves his carbohydrate target of 194 grams.

Top Mistakes People Make When Doing Intermittent Fasting

1) Not eating healthy foods

2) Not drinking enough water

When we fast, our body undergoes cell apoptosis. This promotes cell death and regeneration, which might sound bad, but it's really just breaking down the cells that are not working properly and uses them as fuel. If you are not properly hydrated, the toxins in these cells can't be flushed out.

It's important to note that toxins build up in our fats. When fat is being used as our source of fuel, it is vital that we are stay hydrated so that we can process the toxins through the liver and excrete them. If they are not processed properly the toxins will float around in

the body making us sick.

3) Adding milk to coffees during the fast

Milk contains calories and its enough to set off the

metabolic response. This stops the process of burning

stored energy and causes the body to begin using food

energy.

4) Branch Chain Amino Acids

It might be a good idea to avoid these supplements as

they spike insulin levels and break the fasting process.

Its comes down to individual preference, these

supplements help some people, particularly those who

are just getting start with intensive exercise routines.

5) Not consuming enough minerals

Adding the right kinds of salts to your diet, such as sea salt, during your eating periods is important because our mineral intake can lower while limiting our caloric intake with our mineral needs not being met. The body needs minerals to function correctly.

Remove Sugar As If It Were A Cancer

"The surge in blood sugar and insulin that occurs when you eat any kind of wheat eventually causes an increase in visceral (internal) fat. This fat makes the body more resistant to insulin and increases the risk for diabetes" ~ Dr. William Davis, MD, *Wheat Belly: Lose the Wheat, Lose the Weight, and Find Your Path Back to Health*

In this chapter I am going to be drilling into your head why having an addiction to sugar is a negative way to live. First of all, true power comes from being in control of your emotions. Do you want to be a slave to sugar?

It's normal if you are addicted. Scientists argue that sugar commonly produces stronger cravings than cocaine. Get rid of the sugar, it will increase the likelihood of picking up cancer.

It's just the way life is. Nothings free. Pleasure almost always comes at a cost.

Perhaps the simplest anti-sugar argument is that sugar contains no essential nutrients. Added sugars that come in the form of sucrose or high fructose corn syrup are incredibly calorie dense and come with no nutritional value.

The only benefit of refined sugar is a short-lived energy spike. Beyond this, there is no essential need for sugar.

Many people have a diet where 20% of their calorie intake comes from sugars. This can be very unhealthy in the long term.

We all know that sugar is bad for our teeth, but it isn't just the teeth that suffer. Sugar is harsh on many of our organs. The liver needs to process sugars and break them down into glucose and fructose before digestion.

We don't need a diet that includes glucose because our body produces it on its own.

Fructose on the other hand is not produced by our body and there is no physiological need for it.

The standard person's glucose based metabolic process turns all digested carbs into glucose and depends on the glucose as the main source of fuel for skeletal, brain, and muscle function.

The problem with the body's processing of glucose is that while it a necessary source of energy in low quantities, once it reaches a point of saturation the glucose becomes toxic and will poison the body.

At a biochemical level, glucose plays a necessary role for each cells aerobic and anaerobic processes that produce Adenosine Triphosphate (ATP), the fundamental units of cellular energy. So more glucose allows the ATP to be created with a proportional relationship. However once there is an excess, the cells reach a point of saturation, and the cells are no longer able to handle higher amounts of glucose.

Athe point of saturation, the body is left with the problem of managing this excess of glucose, because glucose becomes toxic when it is left in the blood stream. Studies have shown that glucose is a threat to our immune systems.

Consequently, the body's natural design allows for emergency systems that triggers the storage of glucose in the case of an overload.

Approximately 270 grams of glycogen is stored in the body, 70 grams in the liver and 200 grams in the muscle tissues. This is in preparation for a situation where the blood sugar levels drop too much.

When the glycogen stores are at the full capacity of 270 grams, the remaining glucose will neither be stored in the normal cells or get shuttled away - the only thing left to do with this glucose is to get stored inside of our fat cells.

Continuing to consume more glucose than required to an already over-saturated body is similar to filling a full bath tub with more water. However, the water in the bathtub will pour out while it overflows. In our body's situation, the remaining glucose will get stored in our fat cells and increase our weight.

The other factor to consider in this biochemical equation is insulin.

Our body makes use of insulin as a bridge to transfer glucose from our bloodstream to our individual cells. Our brain's feedback loop recognizes that when glucose has entered the body. When this occurs, the body secretes insulin. The insulin attaches to individual cells and allows for glucose to enter the cells.

When the point of saturation occurs, our body's insulin levels generally remain elevated, even though the cells are functioning at a capacity to eliminate their receptors. As a result, our body has an excess of insulin to combat against the poisonous properties of glucose, but there is still no way to utilize it all.

As time progresses and your body continues to pump even more glucose into an already oversaturated body, our biochemistry tends to create an insulin-resistance. This is known medically as type 2 diabetes. This is because insulin levels have been excessively raised over long periods of time.

So through this you can now see and understand the harmful effects that are caused by oversaturating the body with unsustainable levels of glucose which is likely the main cause of obesity, diabetes, and a myriad of other chronic diseases.

Why Is Glucose So Threatening?

"The doctor of the future will give no medication, but will interest his patients in the care of the human frame, diet and in the cause and prevention of disease." ~Thomas A. Edison

Let's move the evolutionary clock back to a time before the agricultural revolution. This is before there was an abundance of pastas, breads, grains, cereals, and the mass production of processed foods.

In our primal environment, humans thrived mostly on the carbohydrates that came from fruits, vegetables, and fibres. The significant differences between these primal foods and agricultural grain based foods was the differences in caloric densities, which =describes how many carbohydrate calories will be found in each particular food portion.

A single slice of bread will contain about 100 calories and 36 grams of carbohydrates (with 1.5 grams of fibre). A standard sized apple would contain about 100 calories, however it would only have about 25 grams of carbohydrates with a higher amount portion of fibre ~4.5 grams.

What we can draw from these measurements is that the apple has about 69% less carbohydrates but three times more fibre. The addition fibre plays an important role because fibre helps to regulate our blood sugar levels. So although the apple contains a relatively high amount of carbohydrates it compensates for the excess carbohydrates because the fibre limits the damage that an excess amount of glucose can create while it is in the bloodstream.

The contrast between carbohydrate content is even greater when comparing with vegetables. Consuming 100 calories of broccoli would require one to eat at least 3 cups worth, which would only equate to about 17 grams of carbohydrates, but also more than 7 grams of fibre.

So as you can see, it would be extremely difficult for one to reach the required energy or carbohydrates intakes on vegetables alone.

So because of the lack of calorically dense foods found in nature, the biochemistry of the human body did not evolve to handle excessive amounts of glucose because it was difficult to obtain. Unless one was binging on an excess of fruits.

The archaic humans would have to eat an amount large enough to saturate the cellular systems and then on top of that eat the equivalence of 11 more apples to saturate the glycogen stores. This would need to be done for an extended period of time for the body's biochemical responses to change and adapt in order to evade death.

So, as it has become clear, the body was not engineered in a way that is able to sustain immense and consistent intakes of carbohydrates and glucose.

In the modern age, a simple coffee with sugar and cream or a doughnut is enough to completely refill even a depleted glycogen reserve. Consuming cereal in the morning, a sandwich at lunch time, rolls before dinner, and a pizza or pasta as a main course is by no means healthy. But we come from a culture that has

taught us that a lifestyle like this is normal.

Fasted Training

Fasted training is a powerful method for losing weight fast. Like any diet or routine, a level of precaution should be considered to ensure optimal results.

Fasted Cardio

What is fasted cardio?

There is a common misconception that fasted cardio is simply training on an "empty stomach". Fasted cardio is about doing cardio in a "fasted" state. There is a reliance based on the conditions of the body influencing the way your body processes and absorbs the food you eat.

After eating food, it is broken down into a range of molecules that our cells can utilize, and these molecules are then released into the bloodstream. When food is broken down, insulin is released. The insulin's job is to transport molecules to the cells. Insulin levels are dependent on how much food is eaten in a meal. Insulin levels can remain high for several hours.

When the body is breaking down and absorbing food, the body is a postprandial or "fed" state. Once the body has finished processing and absorbing the nutrients, the insulin levels begin to drop again to their baseline level. This is when the body start to enter the "fasted" or "postprandial" states.

Insulin does more than just transport insulin to the cells, it also slows the breakdown of fatty acids. The higher our insulin levels are, the less the body is going to burn fat for energy.

Think about it, why would the body burn up fat if there is immediate energy available in the food that was just consumed? When we eat food, the body holds back from its fat burning processes and uses the energy provided from the meal. A portion of excess energy is stored as body fat for later use.

When our body absorbs and processes foods, the body's insulin levels start to decline which tells the body to start burning fat as a means of fuel. When the absorption of food is complete, the body works entirely from the energy in our fat stores.

So how do we use our body's processes to our advantage when trying to lose weight? Telling some to just work out in the morning when the body is starved, and insulin levels are at a low is not the only advice required for losing weight. The laws of energy balance must still be obeyed with macro intake being monitored appropriately – burn more energy than is consumed.

As mentioned, if ones insulin levels are elevated before a workout, then the body is less likely to break down fat cells throughout the workout (lipolysis will be stunted).

Lipolysis makes up one part of fat loss. The other side of fat loss is based around fat oxidation, the literal "burning" of fatty acids by the cells. The body has the potential to break every fat cell into useable fatty except majority of cells will remain unused. The body can only burn up a finite amount of energy with a portion being reconverted into body fat.

It's important to understand that the totality of fatty acids available dictates the fat oxidation rates. Even though the body might not have the capacity to burn up all of the fatty acids that are mobilized during a fasted cardio session, the more it has access to, the more the body burns.

Studies have shown that the ingestion of carbohydrates reduce fat oxidation while resting and when consumed before physical exercise – you will lose more weight if you don't eat before workouts.

How We Lose Weight

For guys, we generally lose weight on our lower abs, low back, and obliques. For women, generally, fat around the thighs, hips and butt are last places to cut weight. This is pretty common for most people trying to lose weight. It's not a curse, just the physiological mechanisms most of our bodies follow.

This is because the body makes use of chemicals known as "catecholamines", which break down fat cells into useable energy. The catecholamines move through the body and bind with the receptors on fat cells. This then trigger the expenditure of energy that is stored within cells which then enables it to be burned off.

Within fat cells there are two types of receptors for catecholamines, alpha and beta receptors. Put simply, beta receptors accelerate fat mobilization and alpha receptors slow it down.

The more alpha receptors there are within a fat cell the more resistant it will be to mobilization from the catecholamines. On the contrary, the more beta receptors within a fat cell, the more response it will be to the fat mobilizing molecules.

As you might have noticed, the areas of the body that get lean quickly have higher proportions of fat cells with a greater presence of beta receptors than alpha. The areas that have less fat cells also have more alpha-receptors than beta receptors.

The other reason "stubborn fat" remains an issue for people is because of the blood flow distributions throughout the body.

You might have noticed that in areas like the lower back and thighs are colder to touch than parts of the body like the arms and chest. This is because less blood naturally flows to these places.

The lower the blood flow is in an area, the fewer catecholamines there are to reach fat cells which results in slower fat loss.

So there are two factors at place that are a hindrance for dropping weight: large amounts of fat cells that are less responsive to the catecholamines, and the catecholamines are less prevalent because of the reduced blood flow in these places.

This is where fasted cardio comes in:

Blood flow in the abdominal region is increased when you are in a fasted state which makes it easier for the catecholamines to reach the stubborn fat more efficiently, allowing for more mobilization of fat.

https://www.ncbi.nlm.nih.gov/pubmed/17784905

How To Train For Weight Loss

The optimal way for cutting fat and losing weight is high intensity interval training. A study conducted at The University of Western Ontario showed that four to six 30-minute sprints burn more fat over time than 60 minutes of walking on a treadmill. This isn't a once off, it's something that has been consistently proved by many other studies.

https://www.ncbi.nlm.nih.gov/pubmed/8883001

https://www.ncbi.nlm.nih.gov/pubmed/8883001

On top of this, keeping cardio sessions shorter works to preserve strength and muscle density.

https://www.ncbi.nlm.nih.gov/pubmed/19387377

This phenomenon is particularly important when it comes to fasted cardio as it speeds up muscle

degeneration
(https://www.ncbi.nlm.nih.gov/pubmed/12750588).
The more one trains in a fasted state, the more muscle
that is lost.

It is frequently said that high intensity interval training
is performed when fasting is a bad idea since oxidation
rates are lower when doing HIIT.

This is partially true, fat oxidation rates lower as cardio
intensity increases (glycogen is used more readily
instead).

However, research has shown that as we continue to
perform consistent HIIT cardio sessions, the muscles
tend to learn to use lower proportions of glycogen
during workouts, so the muscle cells get consistently
better at oxidizing the fats. This is important because
for someone doing fasted training over time, as HIIT

increases the total amount of fatty acids the body can metabolize in a workout.

Research has shown that HIIT cardio is an effective method for eliminating stubborn abdominal fat as well as the dangerous accumulations of visceral fat. (https://www.health.harvard.edu/family-health-guideAbdominal-fat-and-what-to-do-about-it.shtml)

It shouldn't be a hard decision to make – choosing high intensity interval cardio over something like long distance running. To prevent burn out and muscle degeneration it is suggested for people fasting to do 4 training sessions per week that are around the 20 to 30-minute mark in length.

Fasted Weight Training

Weightlifting causes a significant rise in plasma catecholamine levels, so the mobilization of fat is increased when you are in a fasted state. Therefore, weight lifting is a powerful tool when it comes to weight loss.

If you begin weight lifting in a fasted state, you may find that you feel weaker when making the transition for the first couple of weeks. You may even struggle to do more reps. This is normal. It isn't because muscles are deteriorating. It is because eating a carbohydrate rich meal increases people's performance at the gym.

(https://www.ncbi.nlm.nih.gov/pubmed/19225360)

Once you add the carbs back to your diet prior to workouts, the boost in strength returns.

The body slowly adapts to the fasted state and begins to become more inclined to preserving glycogen stores as well as performance.

How To Increase The Efficiency Of Fasted Training Sessions

Supplements can be a smart idea since they help facilitate the mobilization and burning of fat as well as negate some of the downsides that come with fasted training, since muscle break down is significantly increased during fasted training. The breakdown of muscles tissue is part of the muscle building process, but when too much muscle breakdown occurs, it impairs growth in the long term.

(https://www.ncbi.nlm.nih.gov/pubmed/12750588)

Supplements

A common curiosity among people new to fasting is how supplements should be integrated. First, consuming supplements doesn't always count as fasting. Some supplements have calories and have the capacity to take the body out of fasting mode. Many people are under the impression that vitamin supplements are an absolute necessity when it comes to living a healthy life. When it comes to fasting, people suspect that vitamins are now even more important out of fear. One might think, "When I am eating normally, I need my supplements. I must need them more than ever if I am fasting". It does appear logically sound - aiming to meet the body's needs. But the truth is, autophagy is halted along with the body's natural processes that remove toxins. In short, if things are going into the body, toxins are not being removed.

You might be thinking, "Many vitamins contain 0 calories" – this is true. They won't affect the cleansing process, but its unnecessary and potentially distracts the body form the natural fasting process. If you want to take supplements, take them with your food so that your fasting period can be as pure as possible.

If you are on vitamin supplements for health reasons instead of just as a optimization/preventative measures, then speak with your doctor about it. Ideally you want to find a doctor that is aware and well versed around the benefits of intermittent fasting. Not all doctors are informed and might not see intermittent fasting as something that is beneficial.

Nonetheless, here are the most commonly used supplements for intermittent fasters. Everyone is different and it's worth putting time in when determining which supplements will suit you. Once again, vitamin supplements are by no means a necessity during the intermittent fasting process.

Vitamin D3 Supplements

Vitamin D is produced in the skin in response to sunlight. This is a natural process that begins whenever the skin is directly exposed to sunlight. Another way to build Vitamin D in our bodies is through our diets, as it is also found in many foods. Vitamin D helps regulate the absorption of calcium and phosphorus, as well as maintaining the immune system. It is also vital for healthy development of bones. It's ability to boost the immune system is well documented, and Vitamin D also helps fight many other diseases, such as multiple sclerosis, heart disease, and influenza. There is also strong evidence to show that Vitamin D reduces depression, and conversely, it is common to find that people with depression have a Vitamin D deficiency. Supplementing a diet with Vitamin D has also been shown to help people reduce weight.

Generally, you will be able to make enough Vitamin D in your body if you spend any time in the sun. However, if you are constantly indoors, or always in the shade never in direct contact with sunlight, you can put yourself at risk of a Vitamin D deficiency. If you do spend a lot of time in the sun, be wary of using too much sunscreen. Too much sunscreen can block your skin from direct contact with the sun, therefore creating a Vitamin D deficiency even when you are spending time in the sun. Vitamin D deficiency can result in the person feeling tired, in pain, and generally not feeling well. It can increase the risk of damaging your bones. Long term deficiency can cause a person to constantly be sick, and other health disorders such as obesity, diabetes, depression, chronic fatigue, and osteoporosis.

Excess consumption of Vitamin D can also be detrimental. It can cause your bones to become over calcified, and cause hardening of your blood vessels and organs. Generally, if you are experiencing headaches, dry mouth, nausea, vomiting, or diarrhea while taking large amounts of Vitamin D it is a sign of excessive Vitamin D consumption. It is best to 'grow your own' Vitamin D by spending a healthy amount of time out in the sun daily.

Branch Chain Amino Acids (BCAA's)

β-Hydroxy β-Methylbutyrate or HMB is a supplement that prevents the breakdown of muscles. HMB is a formed when our body breaks down the amino acid known as leucine, this amino acid stimulates protein synthesis.

When an individual is in a fasted state, unnecessary muscle breakdown can occur. BCAA's solve these issues, and on top of that help to fight off feelings of hunger. BCAA's are also 0 calories yet still prevent muscle breakdown. They help keep us feeling full in our fasting sessions. It's worth noting that although they halt feelings of hunger, they do spike insulin levels, which prevents one from gaining the full benefits from intermittent fasting.

Caffeine

Caffeine doesn't need to be consumed in the form of supplements or pills, you can consume caffeine by drinking tea or coffee. Avoid using sugar or milk in your drinks, and you can still maintain the full benefits that come with intermittent fasting. Caffeine helps to suppress your appetite, and beyond this it helps us feel alert and mentally sharp (this isn't just a feeling: studies have shown that caffeine does improve concentration and alertness

(https://www.karger.com/Article/Abstract/118312). Tiredness is one of the downsides that can come in the first week or so of intermittent fasting.

Rhodilia/Roseroot

Roseroot is a herbal adaptogen. Studies suggest that it improves mood as well as mental focus.

(https://www.sciencedirect.com/science/article/pii/S0944711300800550)

It's an inexpensive supplement that is worth experimenting with since it has no side effects and has the potential for some great upsides.

Fat-Soluble Vitamins

Fat-soluble vitamins are the ones that need to be consumed with fat in order for them to be absorbed. If you are going to take vitamin A, vitamin D, vitamin E or vitamin K take them with a meal that contains fat.

Water-Soluble Vitamins

These vitamins are not stored in the body. They are excreted throughout the day if you are consuming liquids. Water soluble vitamins include B-complex vitamins such as B1, B2 and B3. Folic acid and vitamin C are also water soluble. Drinking plenty of water when taking these in order to improve absorption. Consume water throughout the diet to keep yourself feeling full and avoid the build up of toxins.

Coenzyme q10 or CoQ10

CoQ10 plays a vital role in mitochondrial ATP synthesis. It helps convert energy from foods (carbs and fats) and transforms it into the form of energy that our cells use called adenosine triphosphate (ATP). This conversion process that produces ATP has many benefits. For one, it helps us sustain natural energy as well aid in the preservation of muscle mass.

CoQ10 is a vital element for regulating many of our bodies daily functions. It's a natural enzyme that is required by every cell in the body. It is an antioxidant that actually protects our cells from aging. It has been used in medical fields for decades, especially when treating heart problems. Even though the body creates Coq10, a lack of Coq10 is correlated with the damaging effects of oxidative stress also known as free radical damage. A deficiency of CoQ10 has been associated with diabetes, cancer, heart disease, and declines in mental cognition. The body's capacity to convert CoQ10 into its active form called ubiquinol declines with age, especially after age 40. Supplementing with CoQ10 can be especially helpful for those approaching the second half of life.

Creatine

Creatine is a wonderful supplement that is common among weightlifters. Its stimulating effects help keep us focused. In fact it has been shown to increase the function of peoples working memory. Creatine improves the cells ability to produce ATP. Creatine also aids the recovery of muscles.

Fish Oil Supplements/Omega 3

Fish oil supplements contain a small amount of fat which can be enough to alter the fasting process. If you are going to take fish oil during the fasting period limit it to one or two capsules. Fish oil should be consumed during the eating periods. Fish-oil, Krill-oil, or any other omega-3 supplement should be taken with your meals.

Omega-3 fish oil contains eicosapentaenoic acid (EPA) and docosahexaenoic acid (DHA). These acids essential for managing heart disease.

The fatty acids from omega-3 can help to:

- Reduce triglycerides

- Lower blood pressure

- Slow the growth of plaque in arteries

- Lower the probability of heart attack and stroke

- Lower the probability of abnormal heart rhythm

- Lowered chance in sudden cardiac death for people who suffer from heart disease

Omega-3 has also been shown to help brain function assisting children who suffer from the symptoms of ADHD. It is also now used as a preventative for

Alzheimer's Disease as well as a means of managing its effects. The European Journal of Neuroscience conducted a study which showed that fish oil reversed signs of anxiety and depression in fats.

Another reason fish-oil is so powerful is that it is excellent for our joints. Fish-oil has been shown to relieve arthritic pain.

I.F While Traveling or Vacation to Avoid Weight Gain

One of the great things about intermittent fasting is that it can be done anywhere: if you are travelling or on vacation, you are still able to stick to the process of losing weight. The 16 and 8 Rule can be done quite easily by having 2 large meals, one in the morning and one at night time, and the benefits of autophagy can still be reaped.

How Do I Maintain the My Routine While I am Travelling?

Travelling and maintaining any diet is tricky business. The vast majority of restaurants have food options that are often high in refined carbohydrates, which are best avoided.

So, to compensate for the struggles of travel, be prepared. Stay strong and focused.

Here's some tips to help you on your journey.

1) Prepare meals in plastic containers and stored within zip lock bags. Be sure that if you bring any liquids past security that the container size is clearly labelled.

2) Dry foods such as seeds, nuts, and beef jerky are fantastic to carry around at all times.

3) Find stores that sell salads.

4) If you have meals that need to be kept cool, ask at the hotel for a room that has a fridge. If they are hesitant, tell them that you have a severe food allergy and they will likely comply.

5) Keep reusable plates and cutlery with you so that you can enjoy your meal more so than if you were eating with your fingers.

Delayed Gratification And Why It's Important

It doesn't take a genius to figure out that the super successful among us are the ones that make sacrifices and stay focused for long periods of time. As the gurus will preach, "Success is a narrow road". An ideal lifestyle has less distractions, with more emphasis placed on the processes that produce the most results.

The great thing about intermittent fasting is that it increases our self-awareness. We develop a closer relationship with ourselves when we are fasting, because it is uncomfortable and initially we are constantly confronted with our desire to eat.

The discipline achieved through fasting often transfers into other areas of our lives. This is why religions often preach fasting as a means of achieving higher levels of awareness and enlightenment.

Efficiency can be optimized when food is avoided. In fact Elon Musk, arguably one of the world's most hyper efficient entrepreneurs skips breakfast. H wakes up to a Pepsi Max and just works. When he does eat, he eats while working.

From an interview where Elon Musk describes his eating habit:.

"I think it's probably true that having a good breakfast is a good idea, but usually I don't have time for that. Sometimes it's made for me, but probably half the time I don't have any breakfast. I'll have a coffee or something like that.. and a Mars bar, sure.. but I'm trying to cut down on sweet stuff. I think I probably should have an omelette and a coffee or something like that. That seems like the right thing and sometimes I do have that."

Of course, Elon isn't on a diet for optimal health, just for efficiency. Fasting can be achieved easily by not eating during the night and skipping breakfast. This is the approach needed when aiming to build multi billion dollar companies, as well as trying to inhabit other planets: you need to strive for one hundred percent efficiency.

Alcohol And Weight Loss

Alcohol plays an integral role during the leisure time for most cultures. Unfortunately, consuming alcohol is detrimental to our health.

Our ideal diet includes no alcohol, however for some people, avoiding alcohol doesn't feel like a realistic option. There are ways to keep alcohol in your lifestyle and still lose weight.

First of all, the negative effects of alcohol are well documented, from mental impairment, capacity for addiction, liver disease to diabetes. Alcohol affects many of us differently. Some people can live long lives while drinking daily for decades, however, most cannot.

There are probably more reasons to not drink alcohol, than to drink, from a health perspective. Like most things in life, moderation is safer than excess. One of the main problems that comes with binge drinking and adopting a new eating plan is that whilst intoxicated, our inhibitions are often diminished which leads to us eating junk foods in the middle of the night after getting home from bars and clubs.

How Do We Drink Without Interfering With the Weight Loss Process?

Alcohol in its purest form is still quite calorie dense. In every gram of alcohol there is 7 calories.

Nutritionists refer to the calories in alcohol as empty calories – calories without nutritional benefits. When it comes to losing weight, the problem with alcohol is when combined with carbohydrates, fats, and proteins, the fat burning process is postponed which results in greater fat storage.

Robert Atkins, the founder of the Atkins diet – the precursor to the ketogenic diet said:

"Here's the problem with all alcoholic beverages, and the reason I recommend refraining from alcohol consumption on the diet. Alcohol, whenever taken in, is the first fuel to burn. While that's going on, your body will not burn fat. This does not stop the weight loss, it simply postpones it, since the alcohol does not store as glycogen, and you immediately go back into ketosis/lipolysis after the alcohol is used up.

If you must drink alcohol, wine is an acceptable addition to levels beyond the Induction diet. If wine does not suit your taste, straight liquor such as scotch, rye, vodka, and gin would be appropriate, as long as the mixer is sugarless; this means no juice, tonic water; or non-diet soda. Seltzer and diet soda are appropriate."

The benefits of 1 or 2 glasses of red wine are well documented. Red wine is high in resveratrol which is known to protect heart cells from tissue damage after things like strokes. It is also known to mitigate cholesterol accumulation. Beyond this, resveratrol has been shown to relax coronary arteries which help to prevent cardiovascular disease.

A study from Purdue University revealed that red wine has the capacity to fight obesity. A compound commonly found in wines, known as piceatannol which structurally similar to resveratrol has a range of benefits. According to researcher, piceatannol prevents immature fat cells from growing. It has been found to alter gene expressions. This changes the way insulin functions during the fat cells metabolic processes. In the presence of piceatannol, there is an inhibition of adipogenesis – the process of cell growth. What happens is, the piceatannol destroys fat cells in the early phases of development which prevents mass gain. This is because it binds to insulin receptions within fat cells and blocks its ability to control the cells. It also blocks insulin from activating genes that cause fat to form.

Why Refined Sugars Are Your Enemy

Sugar for starters, is more addictive than cocaine. A study performed on mice showed that sugar was preferred over cocaine. Sugar is really good at activating the pleasure centres in the brain to the point where withdrawal can be a legitimate problem when trying to quit.

"Consuming sugar produces effects similar to that of cocaine, altering mood, possibly through its ability to induce reward and pleasure, leading to the seeking out of sugar," according to rodent studies which show that sugar is preferred even over cocaine, and that mice can experience sugar withdrawal.

Added sugar is arguably the since worst ingredient in today's diets.

An excess in sugar intake has a range of harmful effects, from altering one's metabolism to feeding cancer cells. Many scientists argue that constantly having elevated insulin levels can lead to cancer.

Perhaps the simplest anti-sugar argument is that sugar contains no essential nutrients. Added sugars that come in the form of sucrose or high fructose corn syrup are incredibly calorie dense and come with no nutritional value.

The only benefit of refined sugar is a short-lived energy spike, beyond this, there is no essential need for sugar.

Many people have a diet where 20% of their calorie intake comes for sugars, this can be very unhealthy in the long term.

We all know that sugar is bad for our teeth, but it isn't just the teeth that suffer, sugar is harsh on many of our organs. The liver needs to process sugars and break them down into glucose and fructose before digestion.

We don't need a diet that includes glucose because our body produces it on its own.

Fructose on the other hand is not produced by our body and there is no physiological need for it.

Extended Fasts

You might be thinking, why is fasting for more than 24 hours effective?

Let's explore what happens during an extended fast.

For starters the autophagic process is heightened.

At first, many people have feelings of apprehension when they consider fasting. Not eating for an extended period of time is so out of most people's reality, having been trained by society to eat at least 3 staple meals per day, not including snacking. However, once people understand the process and have the necessary procedures to support themselves during the fast, people quickly realise how easy it is. All that is required is a change in mindset, and to understand how our bodies really work.

It takes some time to get used to fasting. In the first few days, the feelings of hunger obviously increase. An effective way to combat these feelings of hunger is to drink more water (but do not exceed your daily recommended intake - too much water can be bad for you). After the second day, the hunger pains generally start to slowly fade away, and many people report experiencing feelings of well-being. The discomfort in the first few days lessens the more experienced you are with fasting as well, as your body adjusts to this new behaviour.

The feelings of well-being experienced may be due to the brain shifting its energy source from glucose to ketone bodies, which are produced through metabolizing fat. There is some evidence to suggest that ketones may help the brain run more efficiently. It generally takes up to 48 hours before glucose levels in the body are low enough for the body to start the process of ketosis, but this can be shortened through exercise, which uses up the glucose faster.

The benefits that come from 24 hour plus fasts can be immense. 24 hours of eating nothing and only consuming water might sound extreme but it very achievable, in fact many people have been able to do more than 30 day fasts for religious purposes and report feeling great because of the fast.

The disciplined nature of fasting enables its practitioners to experience heightened levels of inner strength and confidence. The human body has an incredible ability to heal itself and as well as cleanse itself. Fasting can be hugely beneficial for the body since a diet of only water allows the body to rid itself of toxins. It is important to note that benefits are greater when fasting after eating a diet that is rich in whole foods – a calorie-restrictive diet that includes some chocolates or cheeses will be less impactful compared to a diet that involves splurging on junk foods.

In the first few days, more weight may be loss as excess water is flushed out of the body from the reduction in insulin. Studies on fasting have shown that patients lost weight at between 0.41 to 0.76 pounds per day. This is within the range expected mathematically. Around 2000 calories are burned in a normal day. With a pound of fat containing approximately 3500 calories, an expected weight loss of 0.57 pounds is calculated. The studies on weight loss suggest that metabolism stays stable during fasting, as the rate of calories burned during a fasting period is the same the rate with a normal eating schedule.

Blood levels for all minerals are rarely affected by extended fasting. Electrolyte levels are also rarely abnormal. Occasionally, detected blood magnesium levels are lower, especially in diabetics, but this may be due to magnesium in the body existing within cells rather than in the blood. People who are undergoing fasting are encouraged to maintain healthy vitamin and mineral levels through supplements as a precaution. As imbalances within the body can be dangerous, people with existing medical conditions, such as diabetes, should talk to their doctor prior to starting a fasting program. Fasting should not cause the person to feel faint or unwell (hunger is of course, normal). You should immediately cease fasting and see a doctor if you feel ill, as it may be an indicator that there in an imbalance within your body.

As no food is entering the body, the number of bowel movements will start to decrease. This is normal, as there is less waste to remove from the body. Constipation is an uncomfortable condition caused by a build-up of stool within the body but fasting should not cause this as it is a case of the body not producing stool. The body also recycles many of its own materials from old cells. In the world-record fast, the person fasting had bowel movements every 37 to 48 days.

Short Term Fasts (2-3 days)

In order to gain the full benefits of an extended fast, such as lowered insulin levels and the shedding of extra water weight, you need to fast for more than 48 hours. Patients in fasting studies have reported that the first couple of days during a fasting program have been the hardest, as this is when the body sends the most hunger signals. The difficulty of the fast dramatically drops after the first days as the body begins to release ketones.

That's not to say that short term fasts aren't beneficial. Studies have found that regular short-term fasts can help extend life, regulate blood glucose levels, control lipid levels, and increase weight loss. People who had undergone short term fasts had reduced LDL cholesterol and lower blood pressure. In addition to these benefits, patients gained better appetite control through fasting, which helped the patient gain more long-term benefits.

For people with diabetes or more severe weight issues, a longer fast may be more appropriate for the longer-term benefits, and it would be a waste to suffer through the initial hunger period when the next stage is more beneficial and less stressful.

Medium Term Fasts (7-14 days)

For patients with diabetes, a longer fast is necessary to begin reducing blood glucose levels to a point where ketosis begins. Studies have shown that type 2 diabetes patients are able to reduce their medication much sooner with regular medium-term fasts, as compared to short term fasts. It can take up to 6 days for the person to observe significant improvements in blood sugar levels.

Long Term Fasts (14+ days)

While most studies do not go over the 14-day mark, there are plenty of case studies to suggest that as long as the person has enough stores of energy, essential vitamins, minerals, etc, in their body, they can fast indefinitely. Barbieri's (the world record holder for fasting) 382 day fast is an extreme example of the upper limits of fasting. It is generally suggested that fasting is incorporated into the lifestyle of the individual and used as a tool, rather than for the person to attempt long periods as a standalone treatment.

It's All In The Mind

When we feel hungry, we want to eat. Pretty simple.

Does this mean that we need to eat when we're

hungry? Not necessarily. We have been brought up to

believe that hunger is a signal that our body sends to us

when it is low on fuel, in order for us to eat. While there is a lot of truth to that, another part of hunger is that it is simply a trained response. We have been raised to eat food at certain times in the day, so in certain times in the day we feel hungry. People are rarely hungry when they wake up, even though it has been many hours since they have had food. Yet we are hungry at dinner time, only after a few hours since lunch. Even just smelling some delicious food can trigger feelings of hunger, when you've been well nourished.

In the early 1900s, Ivan Pavlov, a Russian Scientist, was studying digestion in dogs and noticed that dogs would salivate when the bell was rung that signalled that it was mealtime. After this phenomenon was noticed, Pavlov began a series of experiments that showed that after training, a conditioned response can be created in response to a stimulus. The implications of these studies in relation to hunger are immediately clear - we can be conditioned to feel hunger in response to a stimulus. Some stimuli are fairly normal and expected, for example, the smell of food cooking, but others can be completely unrelated to food, such as the time of day. In cases of eating disorders, many stimuli may be working together to create constant feelings of hunger.

When we eat at a certain time every day, we develop a conditioned response to eating at the same time every day. On top of this, as we are purposefully entering into a fast, we will be much more attuned to the fact that we aren't eating. In the first couple of days, when fasting is new, you will think more about food, which in itself can be a hunger stimulus. As we learn to fast however, we will be able to retrain our conditioned responses and become less prone to conditioned hunger, which creates a long-term effect of being more in tune with natural hunger signals. This creates less overeating, as we are not eating based on false hunger signals.

Unless you are underweight or already malnourished, any obstacles to fasting are generally psychological and not physiological. We have learned to eat at certain times, or when we feel certain emotions. In order to break bad eating habits, we must learn to learn to separate false and real feelings of hunger. Fasting can be a great way to retrain our bodies and develop a healthier relationship with food, hunger, and our bodies.

Food Guide

A good strategy to follow is to eat two meals each day. Figure out which portions will suit your macro requirements. The following foods contains approximately amounts of calories.

- o Tuna (light, canned in water, drained, 3 ounces): 101
- o Boiled egg contains 74
- o 1 Egg (large, scrambled): 102
- o Raisins (1.5 ounces): 130
- o Potato, medium (baked, including skin): 161
- o Cheddar cheese (1 slice): 113
- o Pizza (pepperoni, regular crust, one slice): 298
- o Corn (canned, sweet yellow whole kernel, drained, 1 cup): 180
- o Shrimp (cooked under moist heat, 3 ounces): 84
- o Orange juice (frozen concentrate, made with water, 8 ounces): 112
- o Bagel: 289
- o Hot dog (beef and pork): 137

- o Ketchup (1 tablespoon): 15
- o Mixed nuts (dry roasted, with peanuts, salted, 1 ounce): 168
- o Banana, medium: 104
- o Ranch salad dressing (2 tablespoons): 145
- o Peanut butter (creamy, 2 tablespoons): 181
- o Graham cracker (plain, honey, or cinnamon): 58
- o Cola (12 ounces): 137
- o Apple, medium: 71
- o Chicken breast (boneless, skinless, roasted, 3 ounces): 141
- o Pretzels (hard, plain, salted, 1 ounce): 108
- o Beer (regular, 12 ounces): 152
- o Chocolate chip cookie (from packaged dough): 58
- o Granola bar (chewy, with raisins, 1.5-ounce bar): 197
- o Chili with beans (canned, 1 cup): 288
- o Green beans (canned, drained, 1 cup): 41
- o Red wine (cabernet sauvignon, 5 ounces): 124
- o Ice cream (vanilla, 4 ounces): 144
- o Spaghetti (cooked, enriched, without added salt, 1 cup): 220
- o Pork chop (center rib, boneless, broiled, 3 ounces): 222
- o White wine (sauvignon blanc, 5 ounces): 120
- o Salsa (4 ounces): 34
- o Ground beef patty 195 (15 percent fat, 4 ounces, pan-broiled):
- o Potato chips (plain, salted, 1 ounce): 156
- o Spaghetti sauce (marinara, ready to serve, 4 ounces): 93
- o Butter (salted, 1 tablespoon): 103

- o Mustard, yellow (2 teaspoons): 6
- o Coffee (regular, brewed from grounds, black): 2
- o Milk (2 percent milk fat, 8 ounces): 121
- o Yellow cake with chocolate frosting (one piece): 242
- o Oatmeal (plain, cooked in water without salt, 1 cup): 146
- o Jelly doughnut: 288
- o Bread (one slice, wheat or white): 65
- o Rice (white, long grain, cooked, 1 cup): 204
- o Carrots (raw, 1 cup): 51

Eating Healthy And Weight Loss

It isn't the worst piece of advice when people say to have everything in moderation. A diet that is varied to an extent gives us a higher chance of reaching our dietary requirements. However, some foods are worth avoiding. Once again processed/refined sugars have no requirement in our diets – it is in fact quite harmful. As well as this, some vegetables are grown with too many pesticides which makes it best for them to be avoided even if conventional wisdom says they are healthy.

Here is a list of foods known as the dirty dozen according to the Environment Working Group.

Grapes

Bell Peppers

Cucumbers

Strawberries

Spinach

Peaches

Hot Peppers

Cherry Tomatoes

Nectarines

Apples

Celery

Next is the clean 15: the least contaminated fruits and vegetables.

Asparagus
Sweet Peas (frozen)
Sweet Corn (frozen)
Avocados
Eggplant
Mangoes
Papaya
Grapefruit
Cabbage
Kiwi
Cantaloupe
Onions

Mushrooms
Pineapple
Cauliflower

Short list of others to avoid:

Galactose
Carrageenan
Monosodium Glutamate (MSG)
Cereal
Starch (such as white potatoes)

Rice
Maltose
Pasta
Hydrogenated Oils
Corn (syrup, starch, dextrose, dextrin)
Grains

Cane Sugar or Juice
Agave nectar
Sucrose

Guar & Xanthan Gums

The clean vegetables:
Herbs
Asparagus
Mushrooms
Swiss Chard
Shallots
Watercress
Parsnips

Endive
Radishes
Yellow Onion
Butternut Squash
Bok Choy
Turnips
Green Onions
Cassava
Rapini
Mustard Greens
Eggplant
Acorn Squash
Cabbage
Yuccas
Tomatillos
Onions
Collard Greens
Fennel
Seaweed
Spinach
Carrots
Jicama
Tomatoes
Snap Peas
Daikon
Green Beans
Artichoke
Arugula
Chard
Bamboo Shoots
Garlic
Bell Peppers

Turnip Greens
Leeks
Okra
Dandelion Greens
Cucumbers
Lettuce
Squash
Pumpkin
Scallions
Beets
Broccoli and Broccoli Rabe
Lotus Roots
Parsley
Kabocha Squash
Spaghetti Squash
Yams
Sweet Potato
Cauliflower
Celery
Taro
Red Onion
Zucchini
Brussels Sprouts
Sunchokes
Kale

The healthier and cleaner fruits to choose from:

Cherries
Grapes
Plantains
Grapefruit

Avocados
Tomatoes
Dried Version of These Fruits
Passion Fruit
Strawberries
Berries (specifically black, blue, rasp, and strawberries)
Lemons
Cantaloupe
Lychees
Pineapple
Mangoes
Pomegranates
Watermelon
Oranges
Tangerines
Nectarines
Peaches
Apples
Pears
Dates
Apricots
Melons
Plums
Guava
Figs
Limes
Papaya
Bananas
Raspberries

The healthy fats:

Macadamia Oil
Extra-Virgin Olive Oil
Tallow
Butter (grass-fed and pastured)
Palm Shortening (sustainable and organic)
Bacon Fat
Sesame Oil (toasted or cold pressed)
Ghee
Walnut Oil
Coconut Oil (virgin or expeller-pressed for mild flavour)
Duck Fat
Avocado Oil
Lard

Comprehensive list of baking ingredients:

Pure Vanilla Extract
Cream of Tartar
Almond Flour (blanched)
Arrowroot Flour
Dark Chocolate (>85% cacao)
Coconut Flour
Raw Cacao Powder or Cocoa Powder
Coconut Crystals or Palm Sugar
Grade B Maple Syrup
Baking Powder (grain-free)
Honey
Baking Soda

Seeds nuts and butters to choose from:

Tahini
Sunflower Seed Butter
Hazelnuts
Sesame Seeds
Sunflower Seeds
Almond Butter
Pepitas (Pumpkin Seeds)
Cashew Butter
Brazil Nuts
Pecans
Almonds
Walnuts
Cashews
Pine nuts
Macadamia Nuts
Flaxseeds
Chestnuts
Pistachios

Seasonings:

Cilantro
Chicken Stock (recommended) and Broth
Tarragon
Basil
Annatto
Fenugreek
Lavender
Curry
Chervil
Zaatar
Star Anise

Cayenne Pepper
Mace Marjoram
Thyme
Tomato products (Pomi and Bionaturae)
Turmeric
Wasabi
Cardamom
Anise
Liquorice
Chives
Peppermint
Chipotle Powder
Celery Seed
Cumin
Pepper (Black)
Cinnamon
Vanilla
Coriander
Juniper Berry
Bay Leaf
Saffron
Parsley
Spearmint
Horseradish
Rosemary
Galangal
Ginger
Lemon Verbena
Lemongrass
Carob
Paprika
Chili Pepper

Clove
Kaffir Lime Leaves
Mint
Fennel
Dill
Garlic
Sea Salt (Fine-Grained)
Chicory
Mustard Oregano
Caraway

Jarred or Canned foods to choose from:

Curry paste
Organic Tomato Products (Pomi and Bionaturae, diced, strained or paste are great options)
Vinegars (apple cider, pure balsamic, champagne, red wine)
Capers
Unsweetened Applesauce
Olives
Full-fat Coconut Milk
Coconut Aminos
Pickles
Fish sauce (Red Boat brand)

Basic beverages

Mineral Water
Green Tea

Herbal Tea
White Tea
Water
Organic Coffee

Sweets or Snacks

Honey
Dark Chocolate (>85% cocoa)
Carob Powder
Cocoa Powder

How do I maximize my value when shopping?

1) Only shop among the perimeters of the supermarkets. Produce, eggs, meats and dairy and other fresh foods exist here. On the inside aisles the food is likely to be preserved, processed, and more artificial. Always read the labels carefully before buying.

2) Shop at the farmers markets. Prices will be cheaper, you can buy in bulk and you can also

negotiate on the prices. At many markets around closing time you can get larger discounts.

3) Costco and Sam's club can save money too.

4) When buying chicken, bone-in/skin-on cuts of chicken have more flavour and are less expensive.

5) Buy entire chicken and other poultry

How to save time when shopping and cooking.

1) Schedule your meals over the course of the week. Follow the meal plan provided in the previous chapters. When you choose to start trying out different foods, plan out all of the recipes and schedules before going off to buy the ingredients.

2) At the start of the week, cut up all of your vegetables at once and store them in the fridge. Ensure that your knives are sharp.

3) You can re-use any leftover foods later in the week. See the examples set in the meal plan.

4) Make the cooking process simpler. You can stick to foundational meals and mix them up eat time with different spices and herbs.

5) Use a slow cooker. There are many slow-cook recipes provided in the meal plan.

Recipes

Low Carb Pancakes

Ingredients

6 large eggs

10 oz. cream cheese

Salt and pepper

3 tbsp. heavy cream

3 tbsp. butter

3 tbsp. olive oil

3 tbsp. mozzarella cheese

Preparation

Separate the egg yolks from the whites

Grate up the mozzarella

Cooking Instructions

1)Mix the heavy cream, cream cheese, mozzarella and egg yolks in a medium sized bowl, add some salt and pepper.

2) Blend the egg whites in another bowl until it is consistent.

3) Mix the egg whites with the cheese mixture.

4) Melt the butter in a medium skillet over low/mid heat. Place some oil on the pan.

5) With a medium spoon, add 1/4 of the cheese mixture into the skillet.

6) Flip as soon as the base becomes golden brown.

7) Make sure that the cooked ones remain warm until the rest are ready.

Clam Chowder of Kings

Ingredients

1/2 cup celery root or celeriac

1/4 cup celery

1/2 cup yellow onion

2 cups water

1/4 tsp. sea salt

2 slices bacon

1 cups raw cashews

8 oz. bottled clam juice

1/2 sprig thyme

1 bay leaf

 9 oz. can of minced clams

Preparation

1) Soak the cashews in water at room temperature for 3-4 hours before cooking

2) Peel and dice the celery root

3)   Drain and rinse the clams4) Chop up the onion, celery and bacon.

Cooking instructions

1) Cook the bacon in skillet with a cover on medium/high head for 3 minutes.

2) Stir up the onions, celery and celery roots and fry for 10 minutes.

3) Next you add water, clam juice, thyme, bayleaf and salt. Cover it, and allow it to simmer for about 20 minutes.

4) Remove 2 cups of soup from the covered skillet and place it in a blender.

5) After draining and rinsing the cashews, place them in the blender for 40 seconds or until smooth.

6) Mix in the cream with the covered skillet.

7) Stir the clams and allow it to simmer for an additional 6 minutes

8) Once cooked, allow it to sit for 10 minutes so that the soup can thicken.

Roasted Chicken

Ingredients

2 tsp. red-pepper flakes

6 lbs. skin-on chicken (either drumsticks or thighs)

2 sweet onion

6 garlic cloves

1 tsp. black pepper

2 cup cilantro

4 tbsp. apple juice

2 ½ cups basil

½ cup Ketogenic fish sauce

½ cup mint

2 limes

Preparation

Chop up the onion

Preheat the oven to 390°F

Make little wedges out of the limes using a knife

Make a marinate and cover the chicken in it at least 90 minutes before roasting.

Cooking instructions

How to make the marinade

1) Using a blender add in the cilantro, basil, fish sauce, black pepper, garlic, puree of the onion and red-pepper flakes.
2) Place the chicken in a gallon zip-lock bag. Pour in the marinade and squeeze out all the excess air before sealing. Leave in the refrigerator.
3) 30 minutes before cooking take the chicken out of the bag.

Cooking method

1) Line the cooking tray with foil. Put a wire rack on
   top of the foil. Place the chicken in a single layer
   on the rack.
2) Cook for 40 minutes, turn the chicken over at the
   20 minute mark.
3) Serve with the lime pieces.

Steak of the Kings

Ingredients

1 cloves garlic

1/2 sprig of rosemary

1/2 lbs. beef steak

2 tsp extra virgin olive oil

2 tsp balsamic vinegar

1/2 tsp. sea salt

Preparation

Preheat grill to 480ºF

Chop up the garlic cloves

Dice up the rosemary, remove the stems

Mix up the salt, pepper, oil, rosemary and vinegar in a bowl

Place the steaks into a medium sized bowl and allow the marinade to mix in, allow it to sit for 15 minutes.

Cooking instructions

Grill for 6 minutes on each side or to the desired level of brownness.

The Best Breakfast Biscuits

Ingredients

3 large eggs

1 tsp. baking powder

½ tsp. salt

2 oz. flaxseed meal

1 tbsp. butter

1 oz. coconut flour

Preparation

Preheat oven to 340ºF

Add a thin layer of oil to non-stick baking paper

Melt the butter

Directions

1) Mix up the coconut flour, flaxseed and salt in a medium sized bowl.
2) Pour in the melted butter and add breadcrumbs to the ingredients
3) Add in the eggs to the combined mixture and mix some more.
4) With a spoon make separate dollops on the baking paper, ensure there is an inch of space between each one.
5) Bake for 16-19 minutes until golden brown
6) All the biscuits to sit for 5 minutes before serving.

Epic Shroom Burgers

2 tsp. paprika

2 tsp. balsamic vinegar

2 tsp. sea salt

2 cup baby spinach

8 portobello mushrooms

1/2 cup chopped mint

Sea salt and black pepper

6 tbsp. extra virgin olive oil

8 slices red onions (in strips, not rings)

2 lb. ground lamb

Preparation

Dice the mint

Preheat the oven to 390ºF

Preheat grill to 440ºF

Wash the vegetables

Remove the gills and stems from the mushrooms.

Cooking instructions

1) Add a thin lay of olive oil to the mushroom caps and then season with salt and pepper.
2) Place the mushrooms on a baking sheet that is lined with foil. Allow them to roast for 22 minutes, be sure to turn them over at the 11-minute mark.
3) As the mushrooms roast, combine the lamb, mint, paprika, salt and pepper. Shape in to 8 equally sized patties.
4) Cook for 6 minutes on each side.
5) As the burgers cook and the mushrooms roast. Mix the olive oil, salt and vinegar in a small bowl. Pour the mixture on top of the spinach and onion slices. Mix the salad up.
6) On each burger add a layer of mushroom and salad. Serve while hot.

Breakfast Pizza

Ingredients

5 slices pepperoni

2 large eggs

2 slices bacon

Salt and black pepper

1 ounces cheddar cheese

Preparation

Preheat oven to 440°F

Grate the cheese

Directions

1.) Using a medium sized oven proof fry pan, let the bacon cook until crispy.

2.) Separate the fat from the bacon

3.) Cook the eggs in the bacon fat. Add salt and peppers

4.) Bake eggs in the oven for 6-7 minutes

5.) Add cheddar and pepperoni

6.) Allow for the cheese to melt and for the
pepperoni to become crispy.

7.) Once the eggs, pepperoni and cheese are cooked,
remove from the oven, top with bacon and serve.

Beef Stroganoff

Ingredients

1 tsp. sea salt

1 tsp. dried thyme

4 cups almond milk

4 tbsp. apple cider vinegar

4 cloves garlic

4 tbsp. arrowroot flour

4 tbsp. lard

6 cups white mushrooms

2 large white or yellow onion

4 lbs grass-fed ground beef

2 tsp. dried oregano

Preparation

Mince the garlic

Dice up the onion

Slice up the mushrooms

Directions

1.) Place 4 tablespoons of the lard into a large covered frypan with medium heat

2.) Add onion, garlic and mushrooms. Stir until the onions and mushrooms become caramelized, should take approximately 8 minutes.

3.) Once you have removed the vegetable mix, mix in another 2 tablespoons of lard. Add in the beef,

oregano, thyme, apple cider vinegar, salt and
pepper.

4.) Dust the with the arrowroot flour and ensure
that you mix it well enough so that none of the
arrowroot sits in little pools of rendered fat.

5.) Place the vegetable mix into the frypan with beef.

6.) Pour in the almond milk.

7.) Let it simmer on low-medium heat. Leave it
uncovered for 5-10 minutes or unless the sauce
reaches a desired thickness.

Waffles & Blueberries

Ingredients

1 tsp. baking soda

6 large eggs

2 cup raw cashews or macadamia nuts

6 tbsp. coconut oil

1/2 tsp. sea salt

1 cup coconut milk

1 cup blueberries

1 tsp. pure vanilla extract

6 tbsp. coconut flour

6 tbsp. honey or maple syrup

Directions

1) Preheat waffle iron on its lowest setting

2) Using a blender: mix up the eggs, maple syrup (or honey), coconut milk, coconut oil, vanilla extract, macadamia nuts (or cashews), baking soda, coconut flour and sea salt for 1 minute or until it is smooth (this will now be the batter).

3) Add batter to the waffle iron using a spoon until the waffle iron is filled half way.

4) Spread blueberries throughout the batter.

5) Close the lid and cook for 50-60 seconds or until golden brown.

6) Leave the already made waffles in the oven to keep
   them warm whilst the others are cooking.

Low carb Avocado And Eggs

Ingredients:

1 tbsp. fresh lime juice

1 cup cheddar cheese

2 tbsp. cilantro

2 tbsp. butter

2 medium avocados

Sea salt and black pepper

6 tbsp. sour cream

1 clove garlic

4 tbsp. Heavy cream

2/3 small onion

10 large eggs

1/2 jalapeño chili

2 small tomatoes

Make a mixture the day before cooking

Preparation

1) Mix the garlic, onion, jalapeno, avocado and cilantro then add lime juice in a medium bowl

2) Shred up the cheese

3) Skin and seed the avocado and tomatoes

4) Seal the bowl with plastic wrap and leave in the refrigerator overnight. This allows the flavours to combine nicely.

10 minutes before cooking:

Take the mix from the refrigerator

Then:

1) Mix the eggs in a medium sized bowl with sour cream and add seasoning.
2) Melt the butter in a medium sized fry pan and add in the egg mixture
3) Scramble the eggs and then add cheese right before the eggs are cooked.
4) Serve on 3 plates, add salsa and avocado pieces on top.

MEXICAN BACON & EGGS

Ingredients

6 slices bacon

½ a jalapeño

3 ounces red bell pepper

2 ounces onion

Extra-virgin olive oil

4 large eggs

Preparation

Slice up the jalapenos and take out the seeds

Chop the red peppers, onion and bacon

Directions

1) Start frying up the eggs all at once in a medium frypan.

2) In another frypan, add a layer of olive oil, fry up the pepper and onion until tender.

3) Place the vegetables and bacon on a plate, then place the eggs on top and serve hot.

Bacon Meatloaf

Ingredients

2 cup mushrooms

1 cup Pâté

1 tsp. dried thyme

3lb grass-fed ground beef

2 cup onion

20 slices bacon

1/2 cup parsley

½ tsp. sea salt

Preparation

Dice the onions

Chop parsley and mushroom

Preheat oven to 380ºF

Cooking instructions

1) Mix up the ground beef, onion, pate, thyme, mushrooms and sea salt in a large bowl.

2) Once it is consistent, place the mix onto a large
baking sheet.

3) Lay the bacon across the loaf, tuck the ends
under it. Use all the bacon until it covers the
entire loaf.

4) Bake for 70 minutes, using a meat thermometer,
measure when the centre of reaches 165 ºF.

5) Allow it to cool for 6 minutes before serving.

Ham & Slow-Cooked Spinach

12 Large eggs

2 cups of ham

2 cups of baby spinach

½ cup of Greek yogurt

½ cup of coconut milk

1 cup of mushrooms

1 tsp of garlic powder

1 tsp of onion powder

1 tsp. thyme

2 tbsp of coconut oil

Directions

1) Dice up the mushrooms and ham
2) Mix the eggs in a large bowl. Add in the coconut milk, Greek yogurt, salt, pepper, onion power,

thyme and garlic powder. Then add the ham,
spinach and mushrooms.

3) Add a layer of coconut oil to the slow cooker.
Pour in the egg mixture. Cook on high for 2 hours
(or until it sets fully).

VEGGIES & SLOW-COOKED BEEF

Ingredients:

2 small white or yellow onion

2 cup homemade beef stock

8 garlic cloves

2 tsp. dried basil

1 tsp. dried thyme

2 tsp. garlic powder

2 tsp. sea salt

2 cup crushed tomatoes

5 lbs. beef chuck roast

Pinch of red-pepper flakes for flavour

2 tsp. dried oregano

4 cups (400g) carrots

2 tbsp. tomato paste

1 tsp. ground cinnamon

Preparation

Slice the onion

Chop the carrots and garlic

Trim the beefs excess fat and separate the beef into 3-inch chunks

Directions

1) Put the beef pieces in the slow cooker.
2) Add carrots, onion, garlic, basil, garlic powder, thyme, cinnamon, red-pepper flakes and salt.
3) Pour in beef stock, tomato paste and crushed tomatoes.
4) Stir the mixture
5) Then cover the cooker and set on low for 5 or 6 hours.

ASPARAGUS, BACON & CHEESE OMELETTE

Ingredients

1 tbsp. extra-virgin olive oil

6 spears asparagus

2 green onion

4 large eggs

½ green bell pepper

Salt and pepper for seasoning

2 garlic clove

½ tsp. whole grain mustard

½ cup (27g) Gruyere cheese

1 tbsp. butter

2 tsp. fresh parsley

4 slices bacon

4 tbsp. unsweetened almond milk

Preparation

Grate Gruyere cheese

Slice up the green onion

Chop the parsley, asparagus, garlic and green pepper

Directions

1)Cook 4 slices if the bacon in a large frypan. Once it is done, set it aside and slice it up once it cools.

2) Add a tablespoon of olive-oil to the bacon grease in the fry pan. Cook the onion, pepper and garlic until it softens.

3) Mix up the eggs in another bowl. Mix in the almond milk, cheese, mustard, parsley, asparagus and then add in the fried vegetables.

4) Head ½ a tbsp. of butter in another pan, pour the egg mixture on top once it has been heated.

5) Cook both sides of the omelette, ensure that is it cooked thoroughly.

6) Place the omelette on a plate and repeat the process with the other half of the egg mixture.

7) Serve and enjoy!

Chapter 7: Bonus* Workout plans

You don't have to have a gym membership to start

gaining muscle and shredding fat. Body weight training

is a powerful means of getting in shape. The main

benefit comes from the fact that body weight exercises

give us functional strength, they work on multiple

muscle groups simultaneously. One of the problems

beginners at gyms have is that they work out using

machines that only target a single muscle, so the

strength gain isn't actually practical. Gains can be

inconsistent, leaving parts of the body that are weaker and are at more risk of injury.

Bodyweight circuits are extremely effective. Body weight exercises get the heart pumping, works out multiple muscle groups, and burns lots of calories. It burns more calories than cardio alone. Strength training burns calories, and then your body spends the hours after exercising rebuilding the muscles, which burn even more calories – this is known as the 'afterburn effect'.

Before any exercise routine, remember to warm up. Get your heart rate pumping and your muscles moving.

A set of push-ups, jump rope, a light jog or running up and downstairs, are a good way to get started. Aim to move around for about 5 minutes before getting into the high intensity stuff.

Once you warm up here is a routine to follow. This is the bare minimum workout routine you can practice consistently to start seeing results.

30 Jumping Jacks

15 second plank

30 walking lunges, 15 on each leg

15 push ups

25 bodyweight squats

Once you have completed these, do some stretches to mitigate the risks of injury.

There is the natural pain of exerting ourselves as our muscles fatigue, but if you are feeling sharp pains, immediately stop. If you are struggling to get through the entire sets, this is pretty normal, take a few more tries to reach the amount of reps mentioned above.

Gyms are not a requirement for getting into great shape. The process of tearing muscles down and rebuilding them is. Some of the world's greatest athletes don't use gyms. It's not a necessity – nonetheless, it takes commitment for whatever avenue you take as a means of building muscle and shredding fat.

Pull Up Bar

Find a pull up bar. This can be in the form of playground equipment, tree branches or anything high that you can grab onto that will support your weight. Pull ups are a super exercise. If you see anyone who is effortlessly doing pull ups they are almost certainly in great shape. After all, the exercise is requiring us to lift our entire body weight.

Most people skip pull ups because they are so challenging, but the challenge is what gives us our benefits.

Pull ups focus on strengthening the following muscles:

Latissimus Dorsi

One of the main benefits is the back work out that comes from pull ups is the strengthening of the latissimus dorsi often referred to as "lats". These muscles benefit that most from this type of workout. It also helps develop the "v-shaped" look that people aspire for.

Rhomboids

The next major muscle that reap rewards from pull ups are the Rhomboid muscles. The rhomboids are right next to our lats and support them.

Working out the back strengths our core and corrects our posture. One of the major problems people starting at the gym is neglecting their back because they are more focused on the seemingly more superficial muscles which leaves them more prone to injuries. A strong back is foundational for maintaining strength throughout the upper body.

Arm Muscles

Because pulls ups are a compound exercise, they work out more than just the biceps, they work out triceps and forearm muscles.

Abdominals

If you have done pull ups before you will notice that your abs will be really sore the next day. It doesn't seem so intuitive, but oftentimes, pull ups work the core better than sit ups.

Additional Benefits Of Pull Ups:

Beyond this pull ups increase our grip strength, and strengthen our pecs and chest muscles. They work as an excellent means of cardio activity since they will get the blood pumping hard. The nervous system starts to fire up, sharpening the mind.

Perhaps the key reason pull-ups are so great is that they promote more balanced muscle development. The strength training that comes from pull ups has crossover abilities, meaning as your ability to pull yourself up increases so does your ability to push heavy weights.

Pull-ups are so challenging that it is really a battle with the mind, how much can you be pushing despite the pain? When you are tired, how many more reps will you aim to do? Push ups are a very quick way for exhausting our capacities and putting us in the situation where we are forced to increase our mental strength and focus.

Remember, don't give up. Keep trying even if you are forced to do only partial pull ups.

Keep in mind that you can adjust your grips from outside of the bar to inside of the bar, from wide arm span to narrow arm span, all of these variations will change the intensity of the work out and provide you with more exercises.

Get A Personal Trainer When Starting Out

If you can afford a personal trainer, get one. The main problem people have when signing up to gyms is that they struggle to commit to a routine. Discuss your weight goals with your personal trainer and they will help you get to where you want to be. Most of them have seen it all before and know what it takes to lose weight and get into shape. A personal trainer is an excellent way to stay motivated and stay in accordance with your plan.

Many gyms rely on the fact that most people will not use the gym frequently. If everyone was consistent with their health and fitness goals, the gyms would be beyond full capacity. Getting started with a trainer will set you on the right path, prevent injuries, and show you what it takes to succeed. A good personal trainer

will also ensure that you have correct form making
sure you reap the maximum possible benefits from
each work out.

Eventually, the gym becomes a healthy addiction. We
start to feel amazing after each work out and
throughout the week, and our baseline happiness starts
to increase.

Go To The Gym With A Friend

If you have a friend that wants to get in shape, make
each other accountable. It's easier to find yourself going
to the gym in the mornings when you have already
promised your friend that you will be going. Having
accountability throughout areas of your life can help
you maintain discipline and commitment.

Remember To Stretch Or Warm Up

This can not be stressed enough: remember to stretch.

This will help to prevent injuries. Its common sense,

but as they say, *common sense isn't common,* especially

when we are younger. We tend to think our bodies are

invincible. It is only once we start slowing down that

we begin to see our fragility. Stretch!

Congratulations

You are now equipped with the fundamental

knowledge and meal plans that will leave you prepared

for your journey towards becoming the most fit,

focused, healthiest, and happiest person you can be.

Intermittent fasting will help to increase you discipline across all areas of your life. Learning to embrace discomfort is one of the cornerstones for success.

Now the next step to achieving these great benefits begin in the kitchen. Get rid of everything that doesn't serve you, refined sugars and carbs.

The aim is to make it as easy as possible to make the shift.

Now you need to take action and commit to this change right now! Now you are motivated and excited to lose all the unwanted pounds!

So, clear out the bad foods. Don't forget to avoid the inner aisles of the supermarket where all the processed foods live! Be prepared for the impulse items like chocolate bars at the checkout and ignore them. Stick to the pre-prepared shopping list.

It isn't the end of the world if you indulge in some "junk food", as long as you are not surpassing your macro limits then you are in a strong position for losing weight.

It isn't the end of the world if you prematurely break the fast. Its resilience and the willingness to try again that will have ripple effects throughout your life. It's the same grit that brings us back to the pull up bar! You are only defeated when you quit! Keep going, always be pushing yourself to get the most out of life.

As your body makes the shift over the next couple of days or weeks, there may be some dips in your energy levels, changes in mood and some food cravings. These are all temporary and will subside as your body adapts.

If you are tired, try drinking some water or black coffee.

Remember when you are feeling extreme cravings, go back to the tips for fasting section.

If you begin to experience initial mood swings, stay focused on the reasoning behind sticking to this fantastic program. Pay attention to where you will be if you stick to the fasts and be motivated to make positive choices by being scared off by thoughts and fears of where you would be if you don't stick with your diet.

We are creatures of habit and momentum, so stay strong. Be determined, be inspired, and more importantly, stick to the routine!

One of the best ways to stick to your routine is to take an active role on online forums or have a friend or mentor who keeps you accountable to the set routines.

Immerse yourself with great books on nutrition and cut out everything that doesn't serve you.

You will feel proud when you look back and see the difference you have made in your life three weeks from now. You will have changed your entire physique and mentality.

If you have any questions, concerns or would like to get in touch, feel free to contact me at "insert email", I would love to hear from you!

Cheers – To our health

www.ingramcontent.com/pod-product-compliance
Lightning Source LLC
Chambersburg PA
CBHW070116260726
48658CB00001B/122